THE BALNEOTHERAPY HANDBOOK

Bringing Balance Back to Your Body with Balneotherapy's Liquid Solutions and Unveiling Its Advantages

GATLIN ARES

Table of Contents

Introductory

Bathing, typically in mineral-rich or hot waters, is an important component of balneotherapy, which is a therapeutic method that utilizes the practice of bathing for the purpose of boosting overall health and treating a variety of medical ailments. The word "bath" comes from the Latin word "balneum," which also gives us the word "bathroom."

Since ancient times, people have been seeking health benefits from balneotherapy, which is typically associated with spa treatments and health resorts. The water that is utilized in balneotherapy may originate from naturally occurring springs or other mineral-rich sources; alternatively, the water may be manufactured artificially with the addition of minerals.

Both the temperature and the mineral content of the water are subject to change, and it is anticipated that varying combinations will produce varying degrees of therapeutic benefit.

The following are some of the possible advantages of balneotherapy:

• Immersion in warm water has been shown to provide calming effects, as well as a stress-relieving and tension-relieving effect on the muscles.

• Improved Circulation The warmth of the water has the ability to improve circulation, which may be beneficial to the health of the cardiovascular system.

• Pain Reduction: Balneotherapy is occasionally used to reduce the discomfort associated with joint pain and musculoskeletal diseases like arthritis.

• Ailments Affecting the Skin Psoriasis and eczema are two examples of skin ailments that may benefit from drinking mineral-rich waters.

• Disorders of the Respiratory System
Inhalation of steam or mineral vapors during balneotherapy may be beneficial for treating respiratory disorders such as asthma.

It is essential to keep in mind that the scientific data supporting balneotherapy's usefulness for particular ailments might vary widely, despite the fact that certain individuals believe it to be beneficial.

It is best practice to discuss your medical history with a qualified medical practitioner prior to receiving balneotherapy or any other form of alternative therapy. This is especially important if you have any preexisting

health conditions or worries.

CHAPTER ONE
Applications Of Today's Technology

The ancient practice of balneotherapy is still practiced today for a variety of applications related to health and wellness. The following are some of its applications:

• Balneotherapy is a treatment that can be found at many spas and health centers located all over the world. These facilities provide a variety of therapies, including baths in waters rich in minerals, in order to promote relaxation and overall well-being for their guests.

- Rheumatologic disorders: Balneotherapy is frequently utilized as an adjunctive treatment for patients who suffer from rheumatoid arthritis, osteoarthritis, and various other disorders that affect the musculoskeletal system. A reduction in joint discomfort and an increase in joint mobility may result from the buoyancy and temperature of the water, respectively.

- Psoriasis and eczema are two examples of dermatological disorders that may be helped by drinking particular mineral-rich waters. It is claimed that certain waters have beneficial effects on the skin. It is possible that balneotherapy, which makes use of these fluids, will be prescribed as part of the overall treatment plan.

• Inhalation therapy, which may involve the use of steam or vapors that have been infused with minerals, may be of assistance to patients who suffer from respiratory disorders such as asthma or chronic bronchitis.

• Reducing Stress and Contributing to Mental Health and Well-Being Balneotherapy's Capabilities to Relax Patients Can Help Patients Relieve Stress and Improve Their Mental Health. It is well known that soaking in warm water helps to induce relaxation, and it can also be used as a strategy to help alleviate the symptoms of stress and anxiety.

• Individuals who are healing from injuries or operations may benefit from balneotherapy when it is included as part of their rehabilitation regimen. Because of the buoyancy of the water, many workouts can be made easier to manage and less taxing on the joints.

• Recovery after Athletic Competition: Some athletes use balneotherapy into their post-competition routine. After participating in strenuous physical activity, taking a bath in cold water, for instance, is thought to help reduce inflammation as well as muscular soreness.

It is vital to proceed with some degree of caution when engaging in balneotherapy, despite the fact that many people have reported having excellent experiences with the practice.

It is possible that there is insufficient scientific data to support its effectiveness in treating particular illnesses, and individual responses may differ. It is recommended to speak with medical specialists prior to adding balneotherapy into a wellness or treatment plan.

This is especially important to do if you have any preexisting health disorders or concerns that you wish to address.

The Principles Of Hydrotherapy

The utilization of water in a therapeutic setting for the purpose of improving one's overall health and providing relief from a wide range of ailments is what is known as hydrotherapy. The therapeutic use of water is founded on an understanding of the physiological impacts of water as well as its inherent qualities.

The following are some fundamental tenets of hydrotherapy:

• Temperature: In order to achieve a wide range of distinct therapeutic benefits, water can be utilized at a variety of temperatures.

It is common practice to use cold water to treat inflammation and swelling, whilst hot water is known to assist in the relaxation of muscles and the enhancement of circulation. The process of contrast hydrotherapy, also known as alternating between hot and cold water, is intended to increase circulation and speed up the healing process.

• Because of water's buoyancy, the effects of gravity on the body are lessened, making it simpler and less taxing for people who struggle with joint pain or mobility impairments to move around in the water and engage in physical activity. This facility is especially helpful for rehabilitation and exercise for those recovering from surgery or suffering from illnesses like arthritis.

• Hydrostatic Pressure: The pressure that is exerted by water on the body can have a healing effect if it is high enough. The use of hydrostatic pressure has been shown to increase blood circulation and bring about a reduction in edema. People who have issues with their circulation can benefit from this therapy tremendously.

• Viscosity describes the resistance that water presents, making movement through it a laborious process. The resistance from these exercises can be helpful for developing general fitness as well as the strength of individual muscles. Aquatic workouts are used for rehabilitation and fitness goals, and they take advantage of the viscosity of water.

• Surface Tension The surface tension of water enables techniques such as whirlpools and water jets to be utilized in order to produce effects that are analogous to massages. Muscles can be helped to relax, blood flow can be improved, and tension can be relieved in this way.

• Particular Gravity: The human body has a particular gravity that is extremely similar to that of water, which makes it much simpler to move around and find support while in the water. Because of this, it is possible to perform workouts in water that would be difficult or even unpleasant to perform on land.

• Water molecules have both cohesive and adhesive qualities, as demonstrated by their ability to stick together. Wraps and compresses are two examples of therapy modalities that can make advantage of these qualities. For instance, by applying wet compresses to the body, one might infuse moisture and bring about a cold sensation.

• Inhaling steam or being exposed to warm water can have positive benefits on the respiratory system, and both of these methods fall under the category of thermal impacts. In addition to inducing relaxation, reducing muscle tension, and providing a calming feeling, warmth can also help produce relaxation.

The term "hydrotherapy" refers to a variety of treatments that involve the use of water, such as showers, baths, wraps, and exercises performed in the water.

In the treatment of illnesses such as arthritis, musculoskeletal injuries, and certain respiratory conditions, it is frequently combined with other therapeutic procedures and is frequently suggested by medical specialists.

It is vital to seek the counsel of healthcare specialists in order to identify which hydrotherapy treatments are the most suited for an individual's particular needs and problems. This is the case with any therapeutic intervention.

CHAPTER TWO
Composition Of Mineral Waters In A Chemical Sense

Depending on their point of origin, the chemical make-up of mineral waters can display a wide range of variations. Mineral waters can contain variable levels of minerals, trace elements, gasses, and other dissolved compounds.

These amounts can vary depending on the specific mineral water. The following is a list of minerals and elements that are frequently discovered in mineral waters, along with the potential health advantages of each one.

• Calcium is essential for maintaining healthy bones, as well as for proper nerve and muscle function.

• Magnesium is an essential mineral that helps maintain healthy bones, blood glucose levels, and muscle and neuron function.

• Sodium is an essential component for maintaining proper fluid balance, neuron function, and blood pressure.

• Potassium is an element that is necessary for normal muscle and cardiac function, as well as the regulation of fluid balance.

• Sulfate: May have a laxative effect and contribute to the processes of liver detoxification.

• Bicarbonate is an important component in the regulation of pH levels within the body as well as the facilitation of digestion.

• Chloride is essential for maintaining a healthy fluid balance and for the digestive processes.

• It is believed that silica can help maintain healthy skin, hair, and nails.

• Fluoride is beneficial to dental health because it helps prevent tooth decay.

• Zinc is important for immune system function, the healing of wounds, and the creation of DNA.

• Copper is an element that is necessary for the development of red blood cells as well as connective tissues.

• Iron is essential for the transportation of oxygen throughout the blood and the overall metabolism of energy.

• The mineral manganese helps in the creation of bone, the coagulation of blood, and the reduction of inflammation.

• There is some evidence that strontium can help build bone.

• Lithium is an element that can be found in very small concentrations; research has shown that it may have the ability to stabilize mood.

• Iodine is essential for the proper functioning of the thyroid and the generation of hormones.

• Bromide can be found in certain mineral waters, but the consequences of it have not been thoroughly researched.

• Carbon Dioxide is the component that gives some mineral waters their fizz, and there is some evidence to suggest that it also aids with digestion.

It is essential to take into consideration the fact that the concentration of these minerals can be very variable between various brands and origins of mineral water.

In addition, the curative effects of mineral waters are typically attributed not to the action of individual minerals but rather to the synergistic effect of a variety of minerals working together.

People might drink mineral water because they believe it has positive effects on their health, while others might go for particular kinds of mineral water because of the minerals that they contain. However, before making large adjustments to one's water intake, it is very necessary to contact with healthcare specialists. This is especially important for persons who have specific health disorders or concerns.

Different Kinds Of Balneotherapy

The term "balneotherapy" refers to a wide range of different therapeutic treatments, many of which involve taking a bath in mineral-rich or hot waters. There are several distinct forms of balneotherapy that can be utilized to treat a variety of illnesses and promote overall wellness.

The following are some examples of frequent types:

• Hydrotherapy is a broad phrase that refers to any therapeutic use of water. It frequently overlaps with balneotherapy, which is another term for water therapy. The use of water in various forms for therapeutic purposes, such as baths, showers, wraps, and other applications, is known as hydrotherapy.

• The practice of taking a thermal bath involves submerging one's entire body in water of a predetermined temperature, the source of which is traditionally a natural thermal spring. The warmth of the water and the presence of minerals in the water both have the potential to have therapeutic effects, such as the relaxation of muscles, the improvement of circulation, and the alleviation of pain.

• In a manner analogous to that of thermal baths, mineral baths involve the use of water that has been augmented with various minerals, salts, and even gasses. The particular minerals found in the water can have a variety of benefits on the skin and the body, including the treatment of illnesses such as psoriasis and the induction of a state of relaxation.

• Mud Baths: In order to make a therapeutic mud bath, mud or clay obtained from sources rich in minerals is typically combined with water. The treatment consists of applying the mud all over the body, and it is thought to provide effects that are both detoxifying and skin-nourishing.

• Aromatherapy is the use of essential oils for therapeutic purposes, and aromatherapy baths are one form of this practice. When you combine the benefits of hydrotherapy with the possible relaxing or revitalizing effects of specific aromas, as is the case when essential oils are added to bathwater, you get the best of both worlds.

• Kneipp Therapy is a type of hydrotherapy that involves the application of water in a number of different methods, such as treading water, arm baths, and cold compresses. Sebastian Kneipp was a

Bavarian priest who pioneered hydrotherapy in the 19th century. He is honored with the naming of this facility.

• Floating therapy is a form of alternative medicine in which patients suspend themselves in a tank or pool of highly buoyant, often salt-infused water. The temperature of the water is often adjusted to match that of the body, which produces a feeling similar to that of weightlessness and relaxation.

• Bathing with water that has been augmented with salt, often Epsom salt or salt from the Dead Sea, is an example of halotherapy, sometimes known as salt baths. The salt is thought to offer characteristics that are pleasant to the skin and calming to the muscles.

• This treatment combines balneotherapy with light therapy and consists of exposing the body to either natural sunshine or certain wavelengths of artificial light while it is submerged in water. It is referred to as balneophototherapy. Psoriasis is one of the disorders that can be treated with it.

• The treatment known as contrast hydrotherapy consists of alternating between hot and cold water applications. For instance, a person could alternate between taking hot and cold showers or baths to improve circulation and speed up the healing process.

The health goals of the individual as well as their current conditions will determine which type of balneotherapy is most appropriate. It is essential to contact with healthcare specialists, particularly in the case of individuals who already have health difficulties, in order to guarantee that balneotherapy is safe and suitable for the individual's requirements.

CHAPTER THREE
Personalized Intervention Strategies

Personalized treatment plans are individualized healthcare methods that take into account an individual's unique traits, medical history, preferences, and particular health needs.

These factors are taken into consideration while developing a treatment plan for an individual. These programs are intended to give interventions that are specific to a person and highly effective in addressing that person's health challenges.

The following is a list of important aspects and elements to keep in mind when developing individualized treatment plans:

• Medical History: The process of collecting in-depth information about an individual's medical history, which may include past illnesses, surgeries, medications, and the medical history of the individual's family.

• Present Health Status: The evaluation of the individual's present health condition, symptoms, and any previous medical diagnoses that have been made.

• Performing all necessary diagnostic tests in order to collect objective data regarding the individual's current state of health. This could involve a variety of diagnostic procedures, such as blood tests, imaging studies, and others.

• Working together with the individual to determine their desired outcomes with regard to their health. This may include the management of a chronic condition, the achievement of a particular health outcome, or the improvement of overall well-being.

• Developing a treatment strategy that is individually adapted to the requirements and preferences of the individual being treated. Medications, changes in lifestyle and food, increased physical activity, and possibly even other types of therapy interventions could be part of the treatment plan.

• Taking into account the individual's mental, physical, and emotional state of well-being. Personalized treatment programs frequently take a holistic approach, which means that they address a number of different elements of health in order to enhance general wellness.

• Getting the patient involved in their own healthcare by educating them about their disease, the various treatment options available to them, and the significance of following the treatment plan as prescribed.

Patients who are both informed and empowered have a greater chance of taking an active role in their own medical care.

• Putting in place a procedure for the routine monitoring of the individual's progression and making any necessary adjustments to the treatment plan. This may require extra diagnostic testing, additional follow-up sessions, or a revision to the treatment strategy.

• Taking into account and honoring the individual's cultural background as well as their own personal preferences when formulating the treatment strategy. It is necessary to have cultural competence in order to ensure that the individual's values and lifestyle are taken into account while developing the plan.

• Ensuring that all of the healthcare providers involved in the individual's care are working together and coordinating their efforts. This may include primary care physicians, specialists, therapists, and various other professionals working in the healthcare industry.

• Utilizing technological tools, such as electronic health records and telemedicine, to improve the efficiency of communication, monitor progress, and provide more easy access to healthcare services.

• Incorporating preventative measures as well as health promotion methods into the strategy in order to reduce the likelihood of experiencing future health problems.

In this age of precision medicine, when advances in medical science and technology make it possible for therapies to be more precisely targeted and effective, individualized treatment regimens have taken on an even greater level of significance.

The delivery of optimal results and an increase in the overall quality of care can both be accomplished by adapting therapies to the specific requirements of individual patients.

Taking Into Account The Particular Circumstances

When developing individualized treatment plans, it is necessary to take into consideration the unique requirements, obstacles, and features that are linked with the patient's particular health condition. The following are some factors to take into account while designing individualized treatment strategies for particular conditions.

1. Conditions of the Heart and Blood Vessels:

• Taking into account potential danger elements, such as the patient's blood pressure, cholesterol levels, and medical history.

• Adjustments to one's way of life, which may include new eating habits and exercise routines.

• Medication management for disorders such as high blood pressure or high cholesterol.

• Programs to help those who have a higher risk of cardiovascular disease quit smoking.

2. Diabetes:

• Blood glucose targets that are individualized for each patient depending on factors such as age, overall health, and comorbidities.

• Dietary planning, which should include concerns regarding the glycemic index and the counting of carbohydrates.

• Maintaining a consistent monitoring schedule for glucose levels in the blood.

• Medication management, including the administration of insulin treatment or oral drugs.

3. Conditions related to the musculoskeletal system and arthritis:

• Strategies for the management of pain, taking into consideration the kind and degree of arthritis.

• Physical treatment as well as individually designed workout regimens.

• Methods for the protection of joints.

• Mobility aids that can improve one's independence.

4. Conditions Relating to the Mind:

• Psychotherapy or counseling that is individualized to the patient's particular mental health condition(s).

• The administration of medication for the treatment of illnesses such as anxiety and depression.

• The implementation of various methods for relieving stress.

• Social assistance and services available within the community.

5. Conditions of the Respiratory Tract (such COPD and Asthma):

• The recognition and avoidance of any potential triggers.

• Practice with the inhaler technique.

• Rehabilitative pulmonary care for people who have been diagnosed with a chronic respiratory ailment.

• Programs designed to help people who suffer from respiratory problems quit smoking.

6. Cancer:

• Cancer treatment regimens that are tailored specifically to the patient, which may include surgery, chemotherapy, radiation therapy, or immunotherapy.

• Compassionate care for the management of treatment-related adverse effects.

• Support from a mental health professional for coping with the emotional toll that cancer takes.

7. Conditions affecting the nervous system, such as Parkinson's disease and multiple sclerosis:

• Management of medications to reduce the severity of symptoms.

• Physiotherapy, which helps patients improve their movement and coordination.

• Speech therapy or occupational therapy, whatever is more appropriate for the patient.

• Assistive technologies that can improve day-to-day functionality.

8. Conditions that affect the digestive tract, such as inflammatory bowel disease and gastroesophageal reflux disease (GERD):

• Alterations to one's diet in order to alleviate symptoms.

• Medication management for the treatment of inflammation or gastroesophageal reflux disease (GERD).

• Keeping an eye out for and treating any dietary deficits.

• Interventions by surgery if they are deemed required.

9. Disorders of the Kidneys:

• Restrictions to one's diet in order to maintain proper electrolyte and fluid balance.

• Medication management for conditions such as high blood pressure and impaired kidney function.

• Dialysis treatment or a kidney transplant for patients whose renal disease has progressed significantly.

• The management of co-morbid conditions such as diabetes.

10. Conditions Related to the Immune System:

• Medications that suppress the immune system, which are used to manage autoimmune responses.

• Ongoing observation for signs of illness progression and any unintended reactions to treatment.

• Methods of managing pain as well as techniques for enhancing one's quality of life.

• Care that is provided in a team setting by multiple specialists, including immunologists, rheumatologists, etc.

11. Infectious diseases, such as HIV and Hepatitis, for example:

• Antiretroviral therapy as a management strategy for HIV.

• Medication that fights viruses that cause hepatitis.

• Preventative actions and vaccinations to cut down on the possibility of contracting an opportunistic infection.

• Compliance with prescribed treatment protocols in order to achieve the best possible results.

Enhancing the efficacy of individualized treatment regimens for a variety of health issues can be accomplished through collaborative communication between patients and their healthcare professionals, as well as the incorporation of technological tools for monitoring and support.

CHAPTER FOUR
Warnings And Precautions

It is essential in the healthcare industry to take necessary safety procedures in order to protect both patients and healthcare providers. These safety measures are designed to reduce the likelihood of mishaps, injuries, and the transmission of infectious diseases. The following is a list of general safety precautions that are typically taken in contexts related to healthcare:

1. Cleaning Your Hands:

• Washing your hands frequently with soap and water or using hand sanitizers is an effective way to reduce the risk of spreading illnesses. Hand hygiene standards should be followed by healthcare providers at all times, but especially before and after direct patient contact.

2. Personal Protective Equipment, or PPE, includes the following:

• It is vital for healthcare personnel to use personal protective equipment (PPE) correctly in order to protect themselves against exposure to infectious agents and other risks. Examples of PPE include gloves, masks, gowns, and eye protection.

3. Measures to Prevent the Spread of Infection:

• The use of isolation precautions, standard precautions, and any other infection control measures necessary to prevent the spread of infectious diseases within healthcare facilities.

4. Patient Care and Protection:

• Methods for safely lifting and moving patients that minimize the danger of injury to healthcare workers' musculoskeletal systems and cut down on the likelihood of patients losing their balance and falling.

5. Security of Medication:

• Accurate administration of pharmaceuticals, which includes validating patient allergies and performing a thorough review of drug names, dosages, and delivery methods.

• Proper storage and handling of pharmaceuticals to eliminate the possibility of making mistakes and gaining unauthorized access.

6. Identification of the Patient:

• Prior to any medical operation, test, or the administration of medication, the patient's identity must be confirmed by using at least two patient identifiers (for example, the patient's name and date of birth).

7. Prevention of Falls:

• Determining whether or not patients are at danger of falling and taking steps to mitigate those risks, such as installing bed alarms, providing patients with non-slip footwear, and offering aid with movement.

8. Prevention of Fires:

• Knowledge of, and compliance with, fire safety protocols, such as procedures for evacuating the building, using fire extinguishers, and ensuring that all exits and passageways are clear at all times.

9. Security in Electrical Systems:

• The proper usage and maintenance of electrical equipment in order to prevent electrical risks. This includes doing routine checks for frayed cables and ensuring that the equipment is grounded.

10. Codes for Emergencies and Response Procedures:

• Training and drills for handling emergency circumstances, such as cardiac arrest or code blue, to guarantee a prompt and well-coordinated response.

11. Security Concerning Radiation:

• The use of lead aprons and shields when operating diagnostic imaging equipment that produces radiation, as required by the applicable safety regulations.

12. Safety Concerning Sharps:

• The safe and proper disposal of sharps (needles, syringes, etc.) in receptacles that have been approved for that purpose, in order to prevent injuries caused by needlesticks and the transfer of bloodborne diseases.

13. Management of Biohazardous Waste:

• The disposal of biohazardous materials in a manner that is compliant with applicable legislation and guidelines in order to stop the spread of infectious agents.

14. Respect for the Patient's Right to Privacy and Confidentiality:

• Complying with applicable healthcare regulations and legislation, such as the Health Insurance Portability and Accountability Act (HIPAA), in order to protect the privacy of patients and maintain the confidentiality of their medical information.

15. Protection against Chemicals:

• The safe and secure storage, administration, and disposal of chemicals in healthcare settings to reduce the risk of exposure and mishaps.

Many hospitals and other medical facilities already have well-defined safety policies and protocols in place, and their staff members receive training to ensure they follow all of these guidelines. It is necessary for healthcare personnel to participate in ongoing education and receive regular updates if they are to be aware of and adhere to the most recent safety protocols.

Making Your House Into Your Own Personal Spa

Making your own personal spa in the comfort of your own home can be a wonderful way to relax, unwind, and improve your overall health. The following are some suggestions that can assist you in developing a relaxing and rejuvenating home spa experience:

• Find a place in your house that is calm and relaxing, and where you can easily create an environment that is reminiscent of a spa. This might be a restroom, a bedroom, or a room specifically designated for relaxing.

• If you want to make the atmosphere more relaxing, use lighting that is gentle and pleasant. You could want to think about using dimmable lamps, candles, or fairy lights. Stay away from strong and bright lights because they can make it difficult to rest.

• Incorporate fragrances that are calming to the senses. Diffusing essential oils like lavender, chamomile, eucalyptus, or citrus, or using them in scented candles, are both options for using essential oils. There is also the option of using scented sachets or potpourri.

• Make sure that the colors you pick up for your spa are ones that are relaxing. The use of muted blues and greens, along with neutral tones, can help provide an environment of calm. Think about using items like towels, robes, or even decor in these colors.

• Make an investment in comfy seating or possibilities for resting. The coziness of your spa environment can be improved with the addition of a fluffy rug, floor cushions, or a comfortable chair.

• If you want the space to feel like a spa, use materials that are plush and soft. Towels, bathrobes, and blankets made of plush fabric can all contribute to the coziness of your room.

• As background noise, play a curated playlist of soothing songs or recordings of natural environments. On music streaming sites, you can find a variety of spa playlists to choose from. Alternately, the sounds of nature, such as the waves of the ocean or the songs of birds, might help one feel more relaxed.

• If you want to give your spa area a touch of nature, you should decorate with natural components such as bamboo décor, plants, and flowers.

• Include spa treatments as part of your regular regimen. This may involve applying a face mask, exfoliating the body, or taking a nice, soothing bath. Think about utilizing skincare products that are all-natural and calming.

• If you already own a bathtub, you should make it the centerpiece of your at-home spa. To make your soak more indulgent, try including bubbles, bath salts, or bath oils. You might want to think about making use of a bath caddy to keep literature, candles, or a glass of your preferred beverage.

• While you are at the spa, make yourself a delicious smoothie, a cup of herbal tea, or infused water, and sip on them while you relax. Staying hydrated is an important component of self-care.

• As part of your spa regimen, incorporate practices that bring you into the present now, such as slow, deep breathing, meditation, or mild yoga. This might make it easier to relax and might cut down on tension.

• If you want to have a tranquil environment free of screens, turn off all of your electronic gadgets. During your time spent at your home spa, give yourself permission to unplug from the outer world.

Keep in mind that the most important thing is to design an environment that takes into account your personal tastes and preferences while also encouraging a sense of calm and relaxation. Make adjustments to these suggestions according to your own preferences and the amount of space you have available in your home.

Your general health and happiness can benefit from having a home spa environment, whether you use it on a regular basis or just for special occasions.

CHAPTER FIVE
Recipes For Homemade Balneotherapy

The practice of balneotherapy, which refers to the therapeutic use of baths, can be improved with the application of a variety of Do-It-Yourself (DIY) recipes that call for the utilization of natural components. The following is a list of do-it-yourself balneotherapy recipes that you can attempt at home:

1. A Soothing Bath with Lavender:

List of Ingredients:

- A cup's worth of epsom salt
- One-half cup of baking soda
- Ten drops of the essential oil of lavender

Here Are the Directions:

- In a bowl, combine the Epsom salt and the baking soda.
- Mix everything together after adding the essential oil of lavender.
- After adding the mixture to a hot bath, soak for twenty to thirty minutes.

2. Citrus Bliss Bath Salts are the following:

List of Ingredients:

- One cup of table salt
- One-half cup of epsom salt
- The grated rind of one orange and one lemon

- Ten drops of the essential oil of lemon

- A total of five drops of orange essential oil

Here Are the Directions:

- In a bowl, combine the regular table salt with the Epsom salt.

- To taste, add the zest of lemon and orange.

- Mix together the essential oils of lemon and orange after adding them.

- Keep it in an airtight container, and use a half cup of it in your bath.

3. Foot Soak with Minty Freshness:

List of Ingredients:

- A cup's worth of epsom salt
- A quarter of a cup of baking soda
- Ten drops of peppermint oil, a vital ingredient

Here Are the Directions:

- In a bowl, combine the Epsom salt and the baking soda.
- Mix well after adding peppermint essential oil.
- After filling a basin with hot water, pour the mixture to the basin.

- Soak your feet in warm water for about 15 to 20 minutes.

4. Bath Soak Made with Oatmeal and Chamomile:

List of Ingredients:

- One and a half cups of colloidal oatmeal
- One-half cup of chamomile flowers that have been dried (or chamomile tea bags)
- Chamomile essential oil, five drops in total

Here Are the Directions:

- Utilize a blender to reduce the oatmeal to a powder-like consistency.

- Combine oatmeal powder, dried chamomile flowers, and chamomile essential oil in a mixing bowl.

- Soak in a warm bath containing the mixture to get calming relaxation for your skin.

5. Elixir of Rose Petals for the Bath:

List of Ingredients:

- A cup's worth of epsom salt

- A handful of rose petals that have been dried out

- Ten drops of rose oil's key component

Here Are the Directions:

- A bowl should be used to combine Epsom salt with dried rose petals.
- Mix everything together after adding some rose essential oil.
- A delightful experience can be had by adding the mixture to a hot bath and then soaking in it.

6. A Soak in Honey and Milk for the Bath:

List of Ingredients:

- One cup of milk in powdered form
- A quarter cup of honey

Here Are the Directions:

- In a bowl, combine the dry milk powder with the honey.
- An experience that is both nourishing and hydrating can be had by adding the mixture to a warm bath and then soaking in it.

7. Green tea bath for detoxification:

List of Ingredients:

- 4–5 individual bags of green tea
- A cup's worth of epsom salt
- A quarter of a cup of baking soda

Here Are the Directions:

- Steep the green tea bags in hot water for a few minutes, then set the water aside to cool.

- In a bowl, combine the Epsom salt and the baking soda.

- After the green tea has cooled, add it to the mixture.

- A cleansing experience can be had by adding the mixture to a warm bath and then soaking in it.

Make sure that you do not have an allergy to any of the ingredients in any new do-it-yourself bath recipes before you attempt them. In addition, if you have any underlying health ailments or concerns, it is recommended that you speak with a healthcare practitioner. Make use of these do-it-yourself balneotherapy recipes for an at-home experience that is both calming and revitalizing.

Guidelines And Safety Precautions

In order to protect your health and well-being while engaging in do-it-yourself balneotherapy or developing your own spa experiences at home, it is essential to adhere to a set of certain precautions and rules. The following is a list of important precautions and guidelines that should be considered:

• Before attempting any new balneotherapy treatments on your own, you should first seek the advice of a qualified medical practitioner. This is especially important if you are pregnant, have an existing medical condition, or take medication. They are able to offer direction on what is secure and appropriate for the circumstances that you find yourself in.

• Make sure that you are aware of any potential sensitivities or allergies that you may have to certain components, such as essential oils, herbs, or other additives. Before utilizing new components, you should conduct a patch test to make sure you won't have any negative reactions to them.

• Make sure you drink enough of water before, during, and after each of your spa sessions. Because soaking in warm water might cause dehydration, you should make sure to consume a lot of water before and after you do it.

• Check to see if the temperature of the water is appropriate for your wellbeing and protection. A person should avoid drinking water that is very hot since it can cause dehydration and may be dangerous, particularly for people who already have certain health concerns.

• To prevent skin irritation and dehydration, you should keep the length of your baths and soaks to a minimum. A good length of time for a bath is somewhere between twenty and thirty minutes.

• If you want to avoid skin irritation when you get out of the shower, pat your skin dry with a soft towel instead of rubbing it forcefully.

• If you are going to use essential oils in your bath, make sure to dilute them appropriately before you do so. Essential oils that have not been diluted can irritate the skin.

• Preserve the freshness of homemade goods by storing them in a dark, dry area out of direct sunlight. Make sure that the lids are on the containers securely so that the quality of the ingredients can be preserved.

• Before each use, give your bathtub or basin a thorough cleaning to prevent the growth of mold or bacteria.

• If you have any open wounds, infections, or skin conditions, you should steer clear of any do-it-yourself treatments that could make these problems worse. It is recommended that you seek the care of a qualified medical professional.

• Women who are pregnant should exercise caution when using particular essential oils and other ingredients. Before attempting any at-home spa treatments on yourself while pregnant, it is important to check in with a qualified medical professional.

• Stop using the product immediately if you experience any skin irritation, redness, itching, or discomfort while undergoing or after a DIY spa treatment. If the problem persists, seek the advice of a qualified medical professional.

• If you are going to use aromatherapy, pay attention to the concentration of the scents, especially if you have conditions that affect your respiratory system. Make sure that the room has adequate ventilation.

• When handling and making use of ingredients, make sure to follow all applicable safety guidelines. Take handling hot water as an example;

exercise caution and try to prevent spills.

• Your spa area may contain surfaces that are slippery; use caution. For safety's sake, invest in some mats that won't slide around.

Keep in mind that the complexion and overall health of each person is unique, and as a result, the products that are effective for one person might not be appropriate for another. It is always a good idea to start with a small amount of an ingredient and monitor how your body reacts to it. This will help you avoid any unwanted side effects. If you are unsure, it is best to seek the guidance of a healthcare professional or an expert in skincare.

Summary

Balneotherapy can be a delightful and invigorating experience, and so can the creation of a home spa environment and the practice of doing it yourself. Within the convenience of your own home, you can take steps to relax more deeply, improve your overall health, and pamper yourself by adhering to the appropriate safety precautions and guidelines.

When engaging in do-it-yourself spa treatments, it is essential to put safety first and modify your routine so that it caters to your specific requirements.

You might want to talk things over with a healthcare professional, especially if you have any preexisting conditions or worries about your health. When selecting ingredients and fragrances, it is important to take into account any allergies, sensitivities, and personal preferences that the user may have.

The adaptability of do-it-yourself balneotherapy is one of its most appealing features. It doesn't matter if you're relaxing in a warm bath, treating yourself to a facial mask, or practicing mindfulness in a calm setting; the important thing is to craft an experience that is unique to you, caters to your preferences, and helps improve your overall sense of health and happiness.

Don't forget to drink plenty of water, pay attention to the temperature of the water, and stick to the prescribed length of your spa treatments. Embrace a holistic approach and create a truly immersive and therapeutic experience by incorporating elements such as aromatherapy, calming music, and relaxation practices. This will allow you to create the best possible environment for healing.

I wish for you, as you begin your journey of self-care through do-it-yourself balneotherapy, to find moments of peace and rejuvenation, as well as a more profound connection with your own wellbeing.

THE END

www.ingramcontent.com/pod-product-compliance
Lightning Source LLC
Chambersburg PA
CBHW050740260726

48661CB00001B/328